Everyday History

Keeping Clean

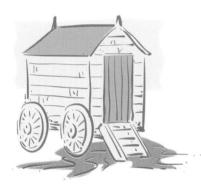

Alex Stewart

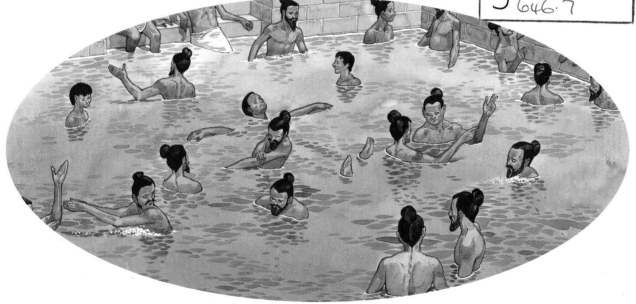

W
FRANKLIN WATTS
NEW YORK • LONDON • SYDNEY

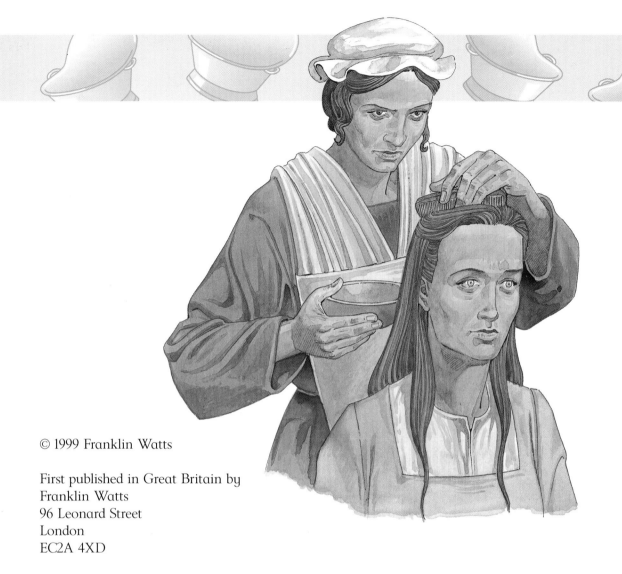

© 1999 Franklin Watts

First published in Great Britain by
Franklin Watts
96 Leonard Street
London
EC2A 4XD

Franklin Watts Australia
14 Mars Road
Lane Cove
NSW 2006
Australia

ISBN: 0 7496 3390 5 (hbk)
        0 7496 3587 8 (pbk)

Dewey Decimal Classification 646.7
A CIP catalogue record for this book is available
from the British Library

Printed in Malaysia

Planning and production by Discovery Books Limited
Editors: Claire Berridge, Gianna Williams
Design: Ian Winton
Art Director: Robert Walster
Illustrators: John James, Stefan Chabluk,
Joanna Williams

Photographs:
4 Liba Taylor/Hutchison Library, 5 Ancient Art &
Architecture Collection, 6 & 7 R Sheridan/Ancient
Art & Architecture Collection, 8 ET Archive, 9 top
Hutchison Library, 9 bottom Peter Newark's
American Pictures, 10 Peter Newark's Pictures, 11 ET
Archive, 13 & 14 Mary Evans Picture Library, 15 top
Corbis, 15 bottom Mary Evans Picture Library,
16 R Opie, 17 Mary Evans Picture Library, 18 Corbis,
19 top Mary Evans Picture Library, 18 bottom Peter
Newark's Pictures, 20 Mary Evans Picture Library,
21 top Mary Evans Picture Library, 21 bottom
Andreas von Einsiedel/National Trust Photographic
Library, 22 top & bottom Mary Evans Picture Library,
23 Corbis, 24 top R Opie, 24 bottom Mary Evans
Picture Library, 25 Peter Newark's Pictures, 26 top &
bottom R Opie, 27 & 28 Mary Evans Picture Library

Acknowledgements:
Franklin Watts would like to thank Jacuzzi UK Ltd
for the loan of material.

Contents

Taking a bath

Human beings have always liked to keep themselves clean. The first people were hunters. Like cats and other hunting animals, they kept clean so their prey wouldn't pick up their scent. They washed themselves in rivers, lakes and streams.

An early bath

The first towns and cities were built about 6,000 years ago. Many were near rivers, so there was plenty of water for drinking and washing. The Sumerians, for example, settled beside the rivers Tigris and Euphrates, and the Egyptians beside the River Nile. Other settlements were built near lakes, wells and waterholes.

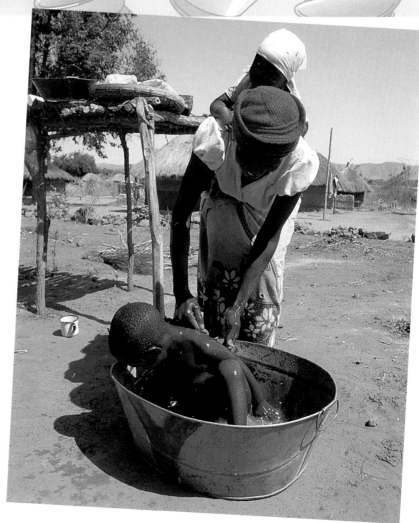

▲ A tin bath helps keep this farmer and her family clean.

Into the tub! Bathers in the Great Bath of Mohenjo-daro about 4,000 years ago.

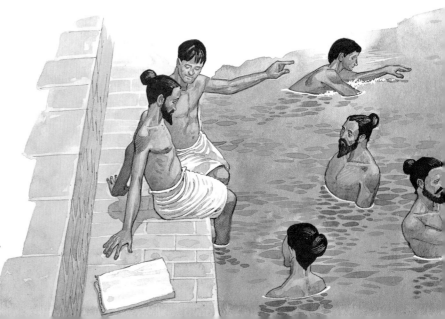

The Indus Valley

Several ancient cities had special baths and bathrooms. Some of the finest were built by the people who lived beside the River Indus. The biggest was at Mohenjo-daro, near Dokri in present-day Pakistan. These early bathing places were very important because washing was a religious ritual.

▲ The remains of the Great Bath at Mohenjo-daro, near the River Indus. The bath was made of brick and sealed with bitumen. It covered 83 square metres (900 square feet).

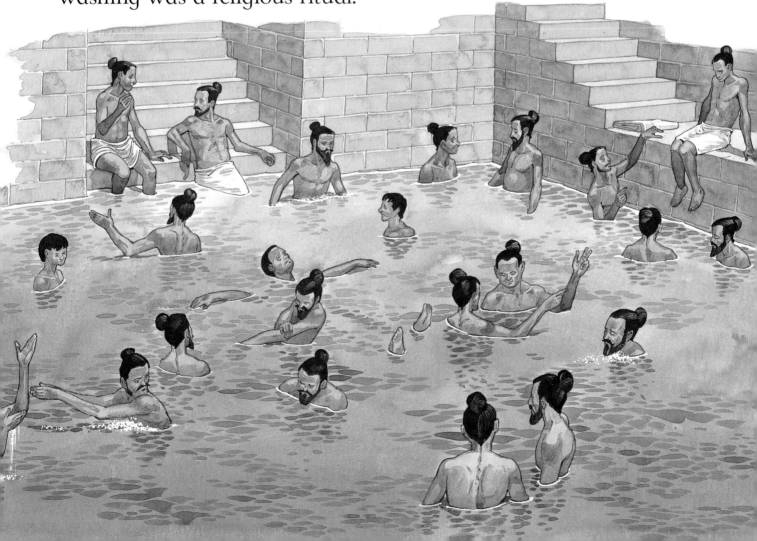

Roman baths

Most Ancient Greeks and Romans liked to keep their bodies clean and in good shape. They took plenty of exercise and built many public baths. Both the Greeks and Romans believed keeping clean showed they were better than other people, whom they called 'barbarians'.

Roman baths were huge. There were rooms for exercise and changing, as well as hot and cold plunges and steam rooms. Some baths also had swimming pools. A Roman could easily spend several hours at the baths, especially as they were popular places to meet and have a chat.

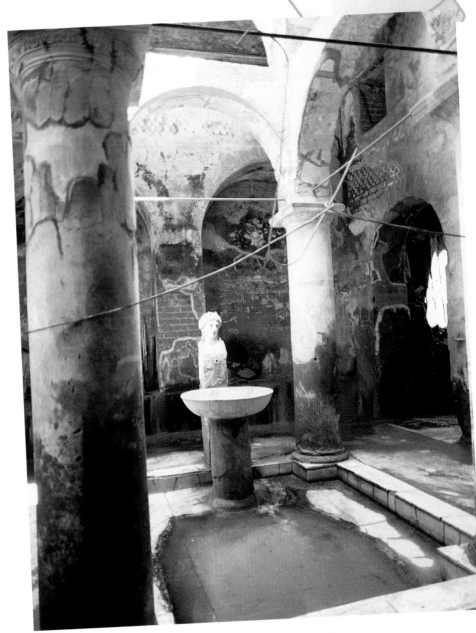

The remains of a Roman bath in present-day Italy from the first century AD.

Scraping clean

Greeks and Romans did not normally wash with soap. After a hot bath, a slave covered them with olive oil and fine sand. This was then scraped off with a metal scraper or 'strigil'. Finally, the skin was freshened up with a mixture of herbs and water.

Scraping yourself clean

You will need some olive oil, fine sand, a scraper and a little clean water.
The scraper can be anything with a flat edge – but make sure it's not too sharp!

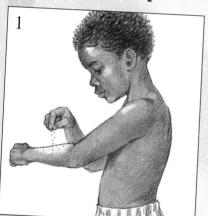

1 Rub olive oil onto your arm or leg and sprinkle some sand onto the oil.

2 Carefully scrape off the oil and sand with your scraper.

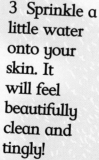

3 Sprinkle a little water onto your skin. It will feel beautifully clean and tingly!

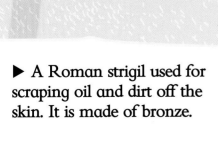

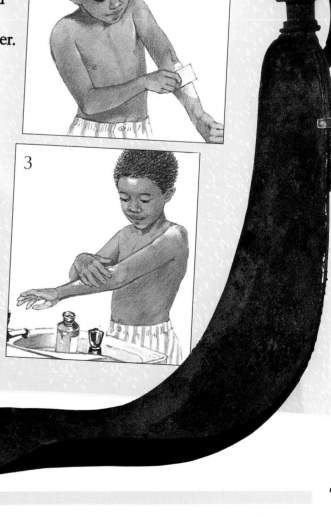

▶ A Roman strigil used for scraping oil and dirt off the skin. It is made of bronze.

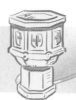

Ceremonial baths

For centuries washing played an important part in most religions. Long ago many faiths started ritual washing or purification. It was thought that cleaning dirt from the body also cleaned evil from the mind.

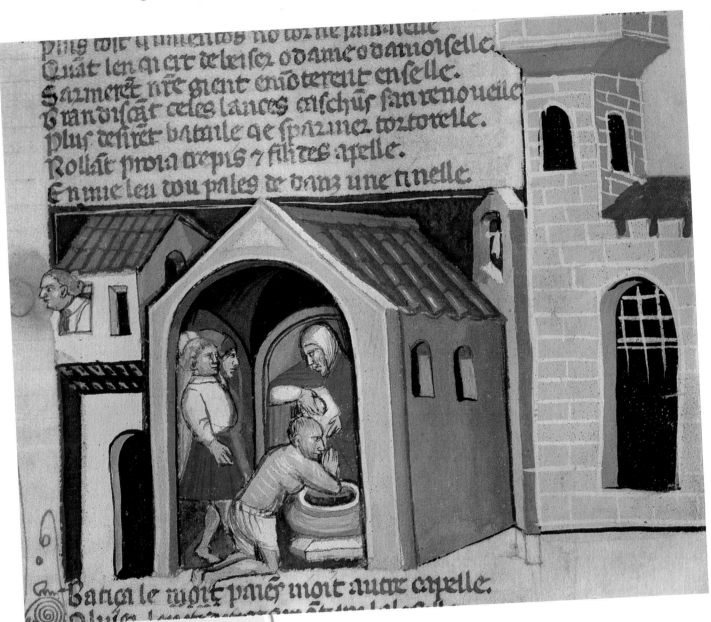

Medieval knights had bathing ceremonies to clean their minds and bodies.

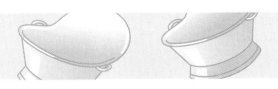

Religious bathing

The Jews purified themselves in a *mikvah*. This was a pool of water, and even more sacred to them than the synagogue where they worshipped. Followers of the Shinto religion had to wash before they visited a holy shrine. Muslims washed before prayer. In India, Hindu pilgrims bathed in the sacred River Ganges.

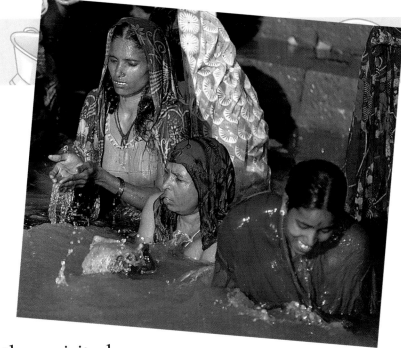

India's Hindus bathe in their most sacred river, the Ganges. Bathing is a religious rite rather than a way to keep clean.

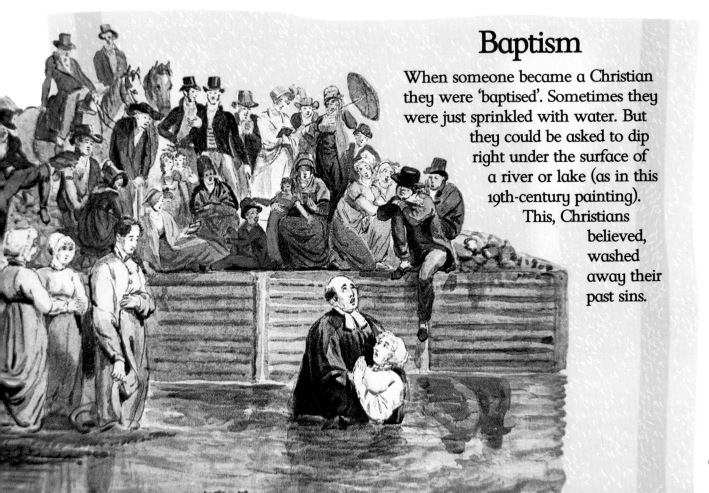

Baptism

When someone became a Christian they were 'baptised'. Sometimes they were just sprinkled with water. But they could be asked to dip right under the surface of a river or lake (as in this 19th-century painting). This, Christians believed, washed away their past sins.

Medieval bath houses

When the Roman Empire collapsed in the fifth century AD, the Roman baths fell into ruin. However, there were still fine Roman-style baths in Byzantium (the eastern part of the old Roman Empire) and in parts of the Arab world such as Baghdad, now the capital of Iraq.

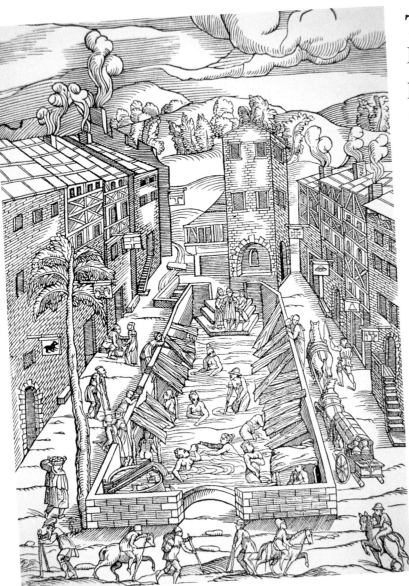

A French public bath drawn in 1553.

The plague

By the twelfth century public baths were again appearing in western Europe. They were not as grand as the Roman baths had been.

But in the middle of the fourteenth century, when the plague hit western Europe, many public bath houses were closed down. People thought they helped spread the plague. Today, we know that keeping clean is a way to stop the plague spreading!

Wooden tubs

Medieval bath houses were found only in towns. Most poor peasants, who lived in the countryside, never had a bath. Wealthy people washed in wooden tubs at home.

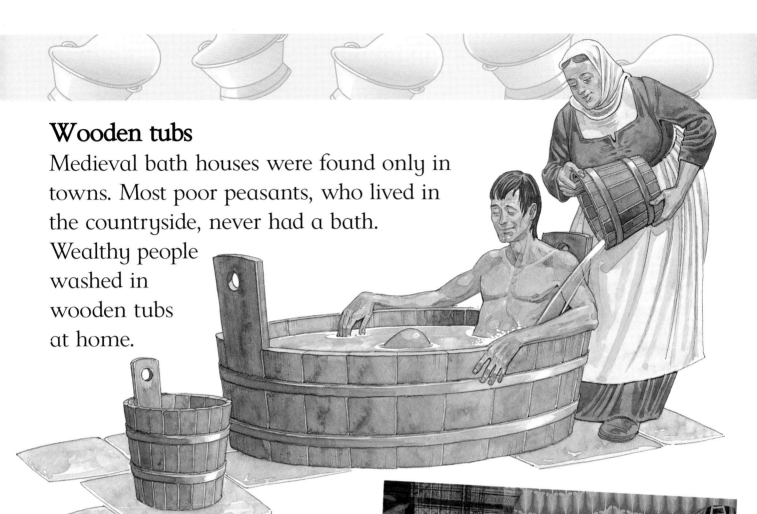

Monks and nuns were expected to keep clean, too. But they did not often wash all over. In fact, very religious people showed their holiness by wearing a prickly hair shirt, which they never changed. When Archbishop Thomas à Becket died, his hair shirt was found crawling with lice — and he was made a saint!

A medieval monk washes a sick man.

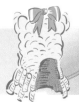

Smells and bugs

Because it was thought that taking a bath could bring on the plague, bathing went out of fashion in the later Middle Ages (1400 to 1600). People's bodies became dirtier. Most clothes were made of wool or leather, and were difficult to wash. As a result, when people crowded together, particularly in a warm room, the smell was dreadful.

Potpourris and pomanders

A pomander

Rich people dealt with this problem by sprinkling scent on their clothes and on tapestries hanging on the walls. Little vessels, called potpourris, were filled with pleasant-smelling spices, petals and herbs. Ladies and gentlemen carried portable potpourris, called pomanders. They were supposed to ward off disease as well as give off nice smells.

Making a pomander

You will need an orange, some cloves and a piece of string.

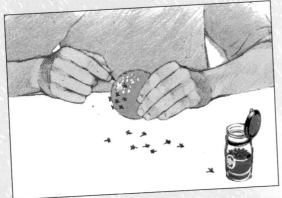

1 Stick as many cloves as you can into the orange.

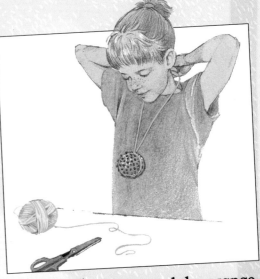

2 Tie the string around the orange and the other end around your wrist or neck. You have made the simplest form of pomander.

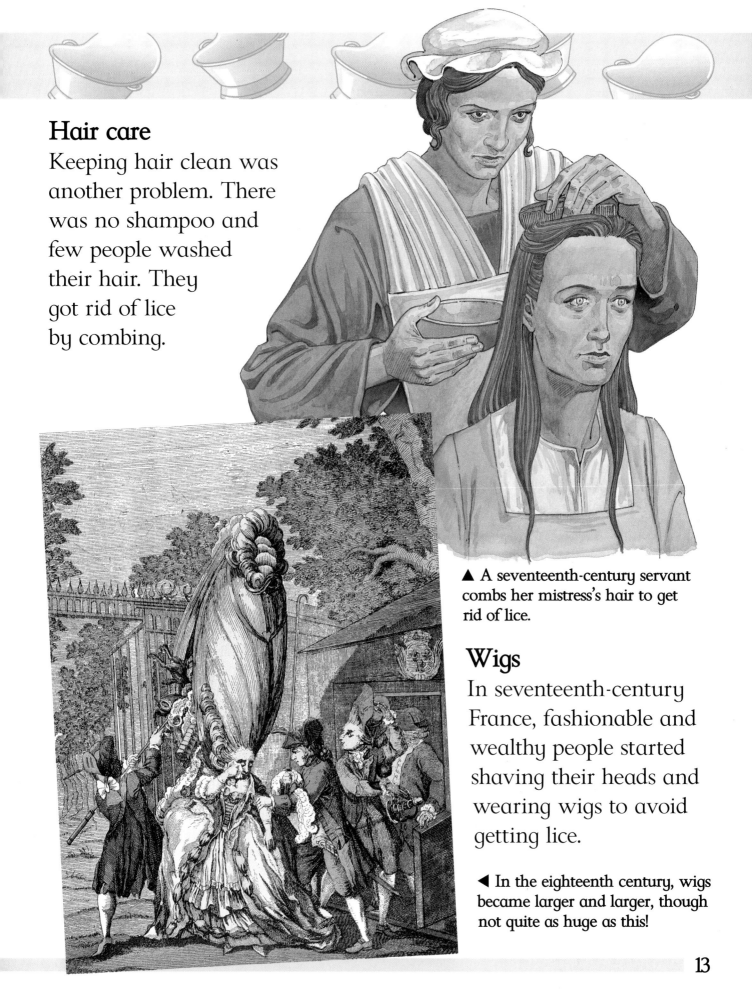

Hair care

Keeping hair clean was another problem. There was no shampoo and few people washed their hair. They got rid of lice by combing.

▲ A seventeenth-century servant combs her mistress's hair to get rid of lice.

Wigs

In seventeenth-century France, fashionable and wealthy people started shaving their heads and wearing wigs to avoid getting lice.

◄ In the eighteenth century, wigs became larger and larger, though not quite as huge as this!

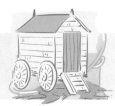

Taking the waters

The Romans, with their passion for keeping clean and healthy, noticed that certain spring waters were good for bathing and for health.

Spa towns

At Bath and Buxton in England, Baden-Baden in Germany and Aix-les-Bains in France, the Romans built settlements with large bath houses around the springs. In the early eighteenth century many of these Roman baths were rebuilt. They became known as spas.

People travelled hundreds of kilometres to visit the spa towns and drink or dip in their waters. The spas where the water was warm, as at Bath, were more popular for bathing.

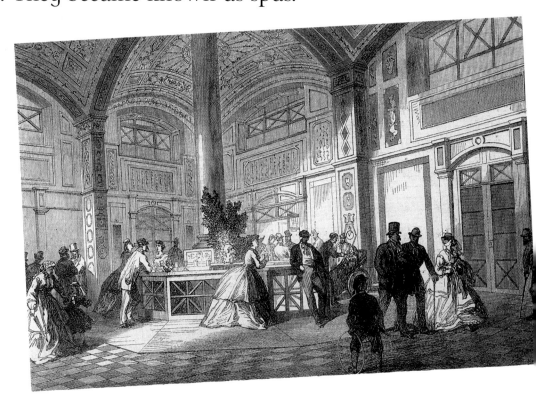

The pump room at Baden-Baden in the mid-nineteenth century.

Other spas, like Vichy in France, produced drinking water rich in minerals. Two of America's best-known spas were Saratoga Springs, New York, and White Sulphur Springs, West Virginia.

14

Saratoga Springs

Native Americans knew that the natural springs at Saratoga, in east-central New York State, were good for the health. European settlers soon became interested in Saratoga, too. The first hotel was built there in 1791, and 50 years later it was one of the most popular spas in America.

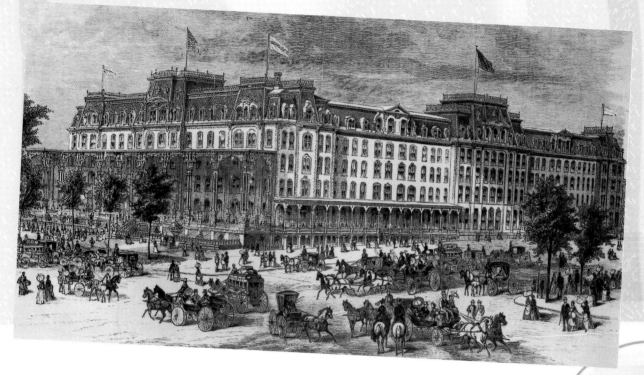

Sea bathing

Since the beginning of history, people living on the coast had washed by swimming in the sea. In the nineteenth century sea bathing became fashionable and seaside resorts grew up all over the world. Sea bathing was good exercise and a cheap way of keeping clean.

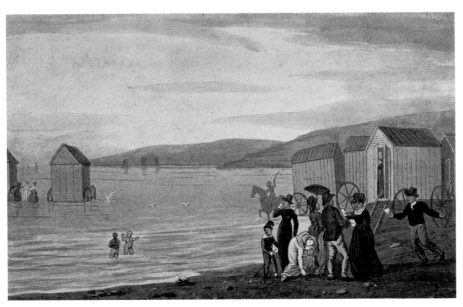

Seaside bathing in Scarborough, Yorkshire in 1813.

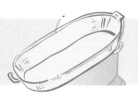

Tin baths

By the eighteenth century the bedrooms of the wealthy had china washbasins on washstands. Maids kept the jugs full of clean water and emptied the basins.

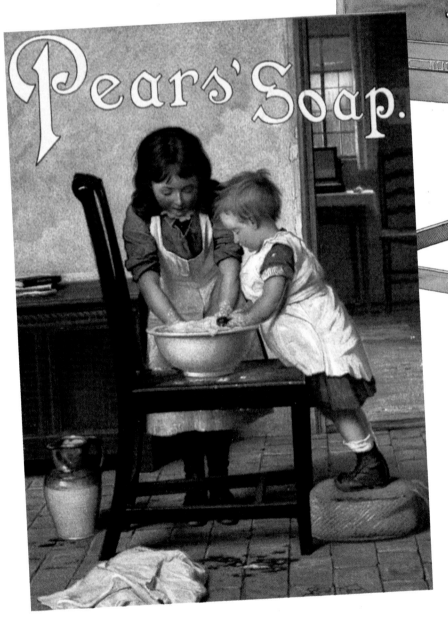

A poster advertising soap in the early 1900s.

Two changes made bathing more popular in the nineteenth century. Doctors discovered that disease-carrying germs lived in dirty conditions. At the same time, bathing was made easier by the manufacture of cheap metal tubs in factories.

Bath tubs

Bath tubs changed the washing habits of Europe and North America. Not many families could afford houses with bathrooms in the nineteenth century, but they could buy a tin bath. Actually, the baths were not made of tin. They were iron sheets plated with thin layers of tin or zinc to stop them rusting.

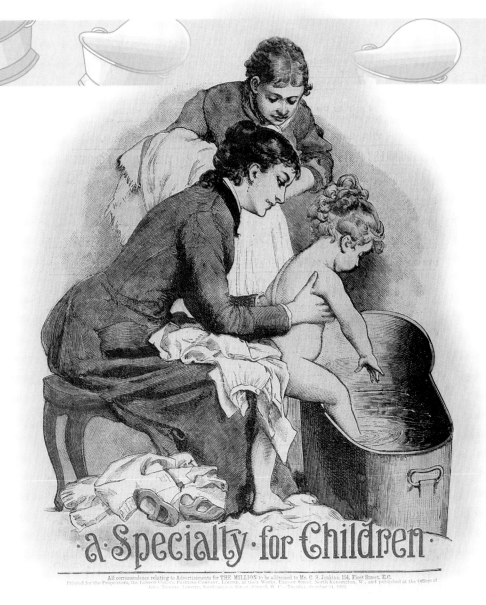

a Specialty for Children

All correspondence relating to Advertisements for THE MILLION to be addressed to Mr. C. S. Jenkins, 154, Fleet Street, E.C.
Printed for the Proprietors, the LONDON COLOUR PRINTING COMPANY, LIMITED, at their Works, Exmoor Street, North Kensington, W., and published at the Offices of
GEO. NEWNES, LIMITED, Southampton Street, Strand, W.C.—Tuesday, October 24, 1893.

Washing in a tin bath, 1893.

Bath sharing

At bath time, the tub was taken out and placed by the fire. The water was heated on the fire or a solid fuel stove, known as a range. Hot water was carried to the bath in a jug or kettle. Because fuel was expensive, hot water was precious: sometimes the whole family bathed in the same water. When they had finished, the dirty water was carried out to the drain.

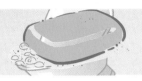

The soap story

The Babylonians are said to have made soap almost 5,000 years ago. The Romans certainly made soap. The first soaps were used for washing clothes. Some were taken as medicine. The idea of using soap to wash the body caught on only slowly. Soaps from southern Europe, made with ashes and olive oil, were best for the skin. The soaps made elsewhere, using animal fats and even fish oil, were often rather smelly.

American settlers making home-made soap on a frontier farm.

Soap tax

Until the nineteenth century, the British government saw soap as a luxury and put a high tax on it. This made it too expensive for the poor to use.

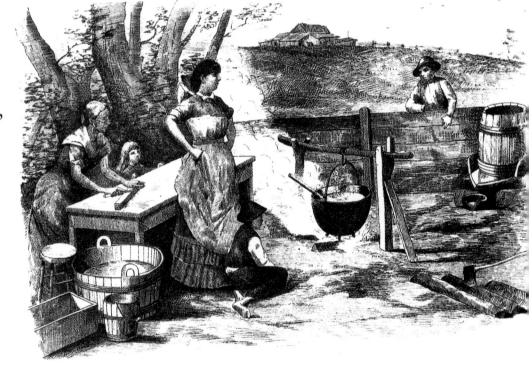

There was no such tax in the New World. American settlers made their own soap. They had good supplies of the right materials: animal fats and timber for making ashes. By the eighteenth century, Americans did a good trade selling purified ashes (known as pearlash) back to Europe.

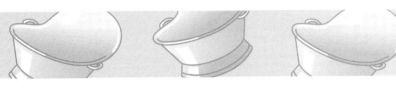

Soap factories

When scientists discovered germs and explained how important it was to keep clean, more and more soap was needed. By the middle of the nineteenth century it was no longer a luxury. Soap-making gradually changed from a handcraft to an industry. Even so, many American homesteaders continued to use home-made soap until well into the twentieth century.

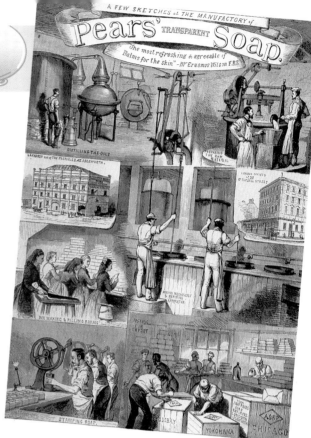

Making soap in the Pears' factory in 1878.

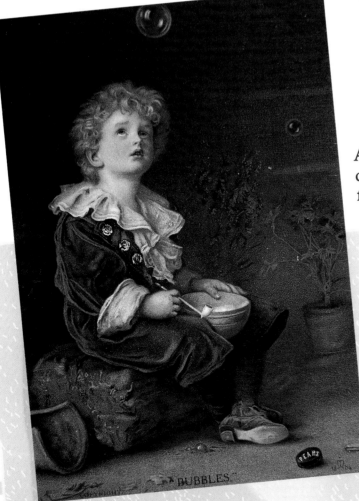

A soap advertisement from 1905.

Bar soap

Home-made soap was soft and jelly-like. It was ladled out of a barrel when needed. Manufactured soap was hardened by adding salt. But only in the nineteenth century did manufacturers start selling soap in wrapped bars.

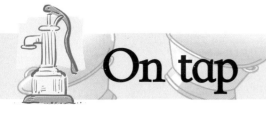

On tap

For thousands of years, water for washing came from rivers, springs or wells. Even in the eighteenth century very few houses had piped water. Many country folk washed outside to save the bother of carrying water into the house.

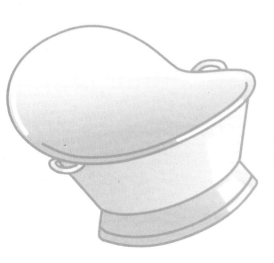

A French water carrier in 1850.

Water carriers

In big cities water carriers went around the streets selling water. When water had to be paid for by the pitcher-full, keeping clean was an expensive business.

Piped water

Things started to change in the nineteenth century, when huge cities sprang up in Europe and North America. Using cast iron pipes, water was brought into the cities from outside. Tanks were set up in the streets, and householders carried the water into their houses and stored it in barrels or buckets.

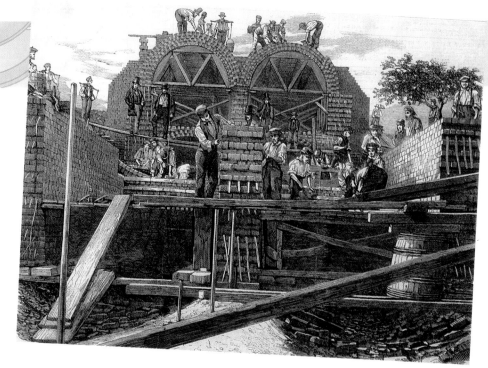

These men are building drainage tunnels in London in about 1850.

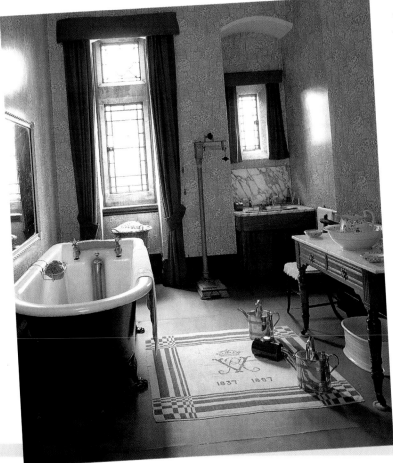

Hot and cold

By the later nineteenth century more homes had their own water supply. Even so, they usually had just a single cold water tap. Only the larger houses had water piped to taps in different rooms. Some had fixed washbasins, usually made of metal, fitted with hot and cold taps and waste pipes.

This Victorian bathroom had running hot and cold water.

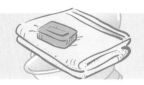

Public baths

By the end of the nineteenth century the houses of the rich had everything needed for keeping clean – running hot and cold water, baths and basins. But the houses of the poor enjoyed none of these luxuries. To deal with this problem, many towns and cities opened up public bath houses.

A Japanese bath house ▶ in the 1800s.

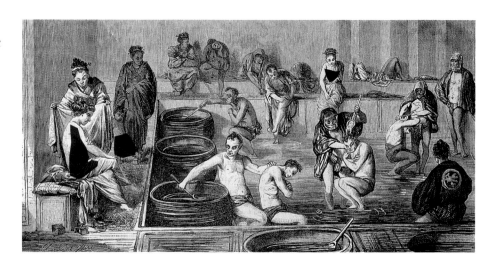

Baths for the homeless

City governments and groups like the Salvation Army began opening hostels for the homeless. Most new arrivals had not washed for days. They had to take a bath before they were allowed to stay. This was to stop them bringing in diseases and bed bugs.

Washing in a poor man's hostel in nineteenth-century London.

Grand bath houses

Some bath houses were on a much grander scale. There were separate bath houses for men and women. The floors and walls were tiled, and the rows of baths were separated by wooden partitions. For a few pence, a man or woman received a towel, a piece of soap and a steaming hot bath. For many customers, this was the only time they ever got really clean.

In 1900 this New York bath house cost five cents to use.

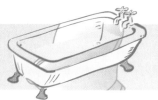

The bathroom

One hundred and fifty years ago it was unusual for a house to have a bathroom. Because they were built for the rich, the first bathrooms were very grand. The fittings were made of marble, polished wood or copper. The maids had to work hard to keep them clean.

▼ Ceramic washbasins became more common in the twentieth century.

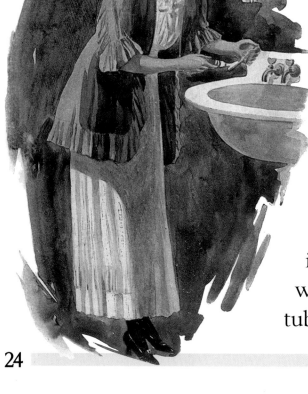

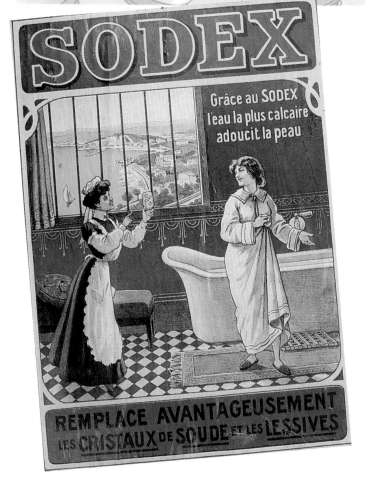

▲ A French advertisement for bath salts, in the nineteenth century.

Ceramic and cast iron

From the 1870s onwards, ceramic (very hard and shiny pottery) was used for lavatories and washbasins. This was much easier to clean than metal. Around 1870 the cast-iron bath tub was invented. The inside was covered with hard, shiny enamel. This type of tub is still found in many homes today.

Building bathrooms

Unlike the old tin tubs, the new cast-iron tubs and ceramic basins were fitted with their own taps. They could not be moved around. So it became usual to build bathrooms in even the smallest and cheapest homes.

Bathrooms were built onto old homes, often at the back. All this took a long time. Even in the 1930s there were still millions of homes in Europe and North America that did not have bathrooms.

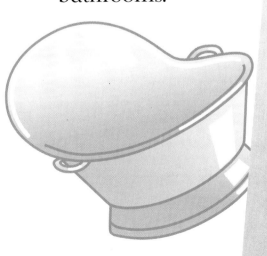

A 1930s American bathroom catalogue.

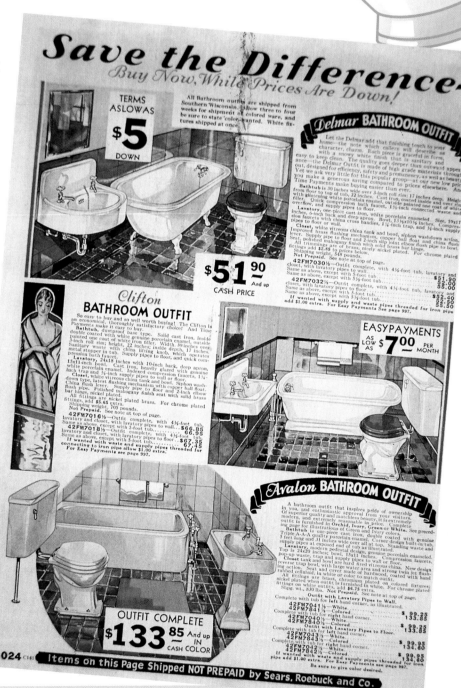

Teeth and hair

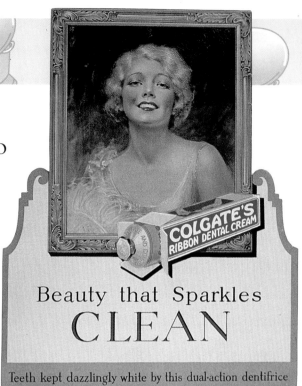

At the time of William Shakespeare (1568-1616), it was quite normal to mention if someone had pleasant-smelling breath. Many people's breath stank! There were no dentists, toothbrushes or toothpaste. The main way of cleaning teeth was with a toothpick.

First toothbrushes

A 1930s toothpaste advertisement.

Horse hair toothbrushes were used in the late seventeenth century. Toothpaste first appeared in the 1820s. Only in the twentieth century did dentists realise the importance of keeping teeth and gums really clean. Toothpastes and mouthwashes were made in all kinds of flavours, and electric toothbrushes cleaned faster and better than any hand-held brush.

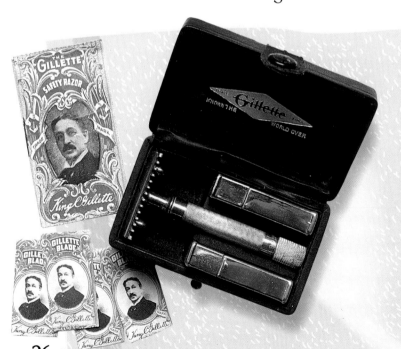

Off with the beard!

From earliest times some men felt they were cleaner if they shaved off their beards. The first razors were made of flint, shell and even solid gold. Steel razors were made in 1740. The American King Camp Gillette began making his famous safety razors at the beginning of the twentieth century. Schick electric razors went on sale in the USA in 1931 and the invention soon spread all over the world.

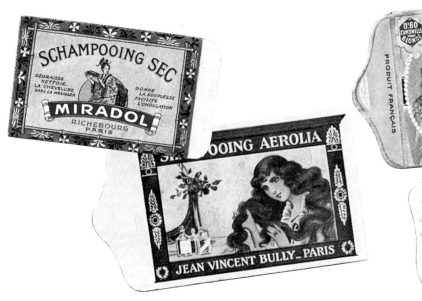

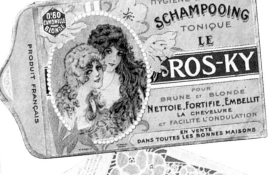

Haircare

Many different types of soap appeared, too. Shampoo was first made in the nineteenth century. In time there were shampoos for different types of hair, shampoos for getting rid of lice and dandruff, and even shampoos with conditioner, perfume and hair-dye in them. At last, hair was clean, shiny and (usually) bug-free!

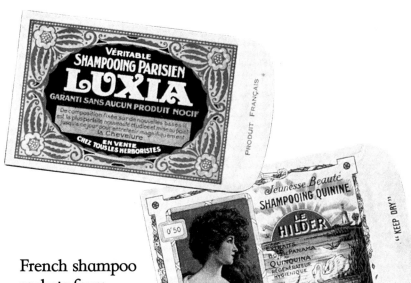

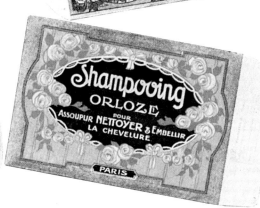

French shampoo sachets from the 1920s.

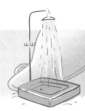

Steam and swirl

In the second half of the twentieth century, new and fun ways of keeping clean became popular. One was the sauna steam bath. This idea may have started in ancient times. It remained popular in Finland, where bathers entered wooden cabins and tipped water onto rocks heated with fire. As clouds of steam rose up, they beat their bodies with twigs to give a fresh and tingling feeling. Outside Finland, modern saunas have the steam but not the beating!

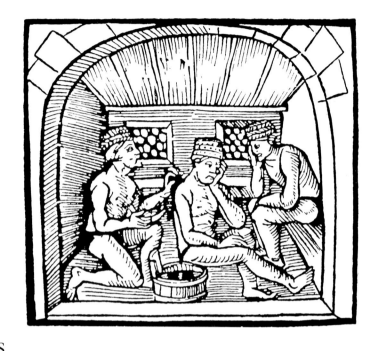

A Danish sauna in the Middle Ages.

Turkish baths

In Turkish baths bathers move from a warm room to a steam room, followed by a massage and finally a cold shower or bath.

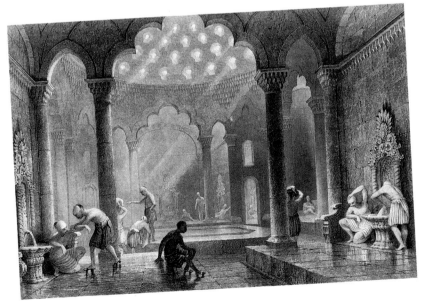

Another type of bath is the Japanese *furo*. After showering in the normal way, bathers stand in a pool of very hot water that reaches to their chest. The water is at least 110° F (43° C).

A nineteenth-century Turkish bath.

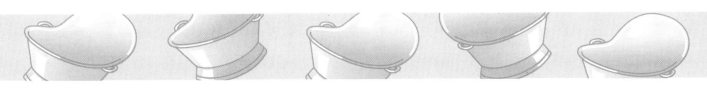

The Jacuzzi

Westerners copied the idea of the furo to make other kinds of bath. One of the most popular was the whirlpool bath, or Jacuzzi.
In these, jets of hot water were squirted into the bath, swirling around the bather.

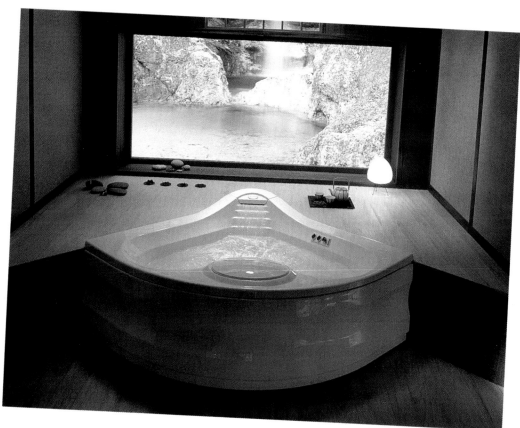

Modern bathing luxury – a Jacuzzi.

Take a shower

Showers also became popular in the twentieth century. Some bathers believed they were healthier than baths because dirty water went straight down the drain. Many other washing aids were sold, too. There were artificial sponges (real sponges had been used for centuries), flannels, liquid soaps, bath salts and all kinds of perfumed bath luxuries. In a little over a 100 years we have come a long way from the old tin bath before the parlour fire!

Timeline

BC

c 3,000	Ancient Egyptians using metal razors.
c 2,800	Soap being made in Babylon.
c 2,500	Great Bath at Mohenjo-daro built.
c 1,700	First Greek bathing rooms built.
863	King Lear said to have been cured by bathing in the waters at Bath, England.

AD

c 100	Most famous Roman baths being built.
c 200	Soap being used in Roman public baths.
c 750	Soap-making starts up again in Italy.
1346	Plague hits Western Europe, leading to the closing of public bath houses.
c 1450	Pomanders in fashion.
1609	Soap-makers arrive in North America.
1624	King Louis XIII begins the men's fashion of wearing a wig.
1770s	Wigs go out of fashion in America.
1790s	Toothbrush made.
1791	First hotel built at Saratoga Springs, New York.
1820s	Hot water being piped around houses. Shampoo first made. Toothpaste first made.
1828	First safety razor made in Sheffield, England.
1853	British soap tax abolished.
1870	Cast-iron bath tubs made in England.
1870s	Thomas Twyford makes ceramic bathroom fittings.
c 1901	Gillette begins making safety razors.
1931	First successful electric razor on the market.
c 1960	First stainless steel razor blade mad
1968	American Roy Jacuzzi invents whirlpool bath.

Glossary

Antiseptic Germ-killer.

Bitumen Black, sticky, waterproof substance.

Ceramic Very hard pottery.

Conditioner Something that makes hair look shiny and stay in place.

Enamel Tough, shiny, non-rusting coating for metal.

Furo Very hot Japanese bath.

Manufacture Make.

Medieval Something from the 'Middle Ages'.

Middle Ages Period of European history from about AD 1000 − 1450.

Monastery House where monks live and pray.

Pearlash Purified wood ash.

Plague The killer disease spread by fleas.

Pomander Hand-held 'potpourri'.

Portable Able to be carried about.

Potpourri Box with holes in it holding sweet-smelling dried flowers, spices, etc.

Purification Making pure.

Resort Place where people go for holidays.

Rite Religious custom.

Sauna Steam bath.

Spa Place famous for its healthy waters.

Strigil Body scraper.

Tapestry Woven cloth for hanging on the wall.

Further reading

Bryant-Mole, Karen, *Keeping Clean (History From Objects)*, Wayland, 1996

Kerr, Daisy, *Keeping Clean (A Very Peculiar History)*, Franklin Watts, 1995

Index
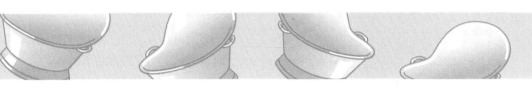